THE SIMPLE MIRACLE CURE

A HEALING EXERCISE FOR CANCER

BY: JOHN MARCOLA

Contents

Disclaimer

The information provided in this book, "The Simple Miracle Cure: A Healing Exercise for Cancer" is intended for educational purposes only. It is not intended to be a substitute for professional medical advice, diagnosis, or treatment.

The content of this book is based on research, personal experience, and the experiences of others who have shared their stories. While every effort has been made to ensure the accuracy and completeness of the information presented, the author and publisher do not guarantee the effectiveness or safety of any treatment, supplement, or dietary advice discussed.

Cancer treatment is a complex and individualized process that should be overseen by qualified healthcare professionals. Readers are strongly advised to consult with their healthcare provider before making any changes to their treatment plan or lifestyle based on the information provided in this book.

The author and publisher disclaim any liability for any adverse effects or consequences resulting from the use or application of the information contained in this book. The decision to use the information in this book is solely at the risk of the reader/patient.

It is important to remember that each person's body and health circumstances are unique. What works for one individual may not work for another. It is always best to seek personalized medical advice and care from a qualified healthcare professional.

BOOKS WRITTEN BY THE SAME AUTHOR:

* BID FAREWELL TO GIARDIASIS

* BID FAREWELL TO HERPES

* BID FAREWELL TO CROHN'S DISEASE

* THE VITAL ELEMENTS OF WELLNESS FOR HEALING CANCER: EARTH, WATER, FIRE, AND ETHER.

* THE TURPENTINE HEALING BATH

* TB, OR NOT TB: NURTURING NATURE'S CURE: TRIUMPH OVER TUBERCULOSIS

* THE TRICK AGAINST TRICH: BID FAREWELL TO TRICHOMONIASIS NATURALLY

* THE CURE OF BLASTOCYSTIS.HOMINIS

* HIATAL HERNIA HEALING MADE SIMPLE: GEORGIA KNAPP APPROACH

* ENGINEERING VITALITY: THE NISHI-KNAP BLUEPRINT FOR HEALTH AND REJUVENATION

* VITALITY OIL CHANGE: YOUR BODY'S DETOX GUIDE AND PROTOCOL

* <u>BED BUGS BE GONE</u>: THE ULTIMATE GUIDE TO NATURAL

EXTERMINATION OF THESE MICRO-VAMPIRES

* <u>RECLAIMING HOMO ERECTUS</u>: THE SELF-CHIROPRACTIC HEALING

GUIDE TO UPRIGHT LIVING

* <u>BID FAREWELL TO AMOEBIASIS</u>

* <u>NATUROPATHIC APPROACH TO ELIMINATING PERSISTENT

VIRAL INFECTIONS</u>: A COMPREHENSIVE PROTOCOL

* <u>MASTERING CANADIAN PHARMACIST EVALUATION EXAM:

PART 1</u> - CONQUERING MCQ EVALUATION EXAMS

* <u>HEALING THE HAZE: A GUIDE TO BENZO AND BARBITURATE

WITHDRAWAL</u>

* <u>MISLEAD BY LEAD</u>: UNRAVELING THE DETOXIFICATION SOLUTION

FOR LEAD POISONING

Introduction

This concise booklet introduces a powerful tool for effectively

combating cancer, drawing on the insights of renowned practitioners

such as Dr. Max Gerson, Katsuzo Nishi, and Dr. Lobrey. The exercise

described is not only refreshing but also vitalizing, offering both

preventive and therapeutic benefits against cancer. Persistence is key,

as long-term commitment to this exercise can yield remarkable results.

Katsuzo Nishi's work highlights numerous cancer patients who, having

been given terminal diagnoses by their physicians, successfully

recovered through regular practice of this exercise. Similarly, Russian journalist Maya Gugulan overcame cancer, which had persisted despite three failed chemotherapy treatments, by adhering to a strict, healthy diet and incorporating this exercise into her routine. The exercise is exceptionally safe, unlike other airbath exercises that may induce or exacerbate cold symptoms. In fact, it can expedite recovery from a cold if practiced during illness.

This exercise serves as a potent detoxification tool, functioning as a form of skin gymnastics that promotes venous return of blood to the heart. This stimulation benefits the liver and can be beneficial for various ailments beyond cancer, including digestive issues, colonic pain, skin disorders, mental health concerns, and infections. By flooding the body with fresh air and oxygen, this exercise revitalizes and rejuvenates, aiding the body in eliminating toxic gases through the skin, akin to the role of the lungs.

The Emperor of Maladies

Cancer, often referred to as the "emperor of maladies," is on the rise and is projected to become the leading cause of mortality in many nations, surpassing even cardiovascular diseases and diabetes. Alarmingly, research indicates that we may face a tsunami of cancer cases in the coming decades. According to the World Health Organization, over 35 million new cancer cases are predicted in 2050, representing a 77% increase from the estimated 20 million cases in 2022. This impending crisis underscores the urgent need for effective solutions to combat cancer.

While the pharmaceutical industry has developed some promising treatments, such as immunotherapy, it is crucial to address the underlying issues rather than simply treating the symptoms. Immunotherapy, for example, aims to boost the immune system's ability to fight cancer, but it may be ineffective if the immune system is already compromised or overburdened by toxins. In such cases, detoxification of the body may be necessary before attempting to stimulate the immune system.

It is essential to seek comprehensive solutions that address the root causes of cancer rather than relying solely on symptomatic treatments. By focusing on detoxification and supporting the body's natural defenses, we can work towards more effective and lasting solutions for combating this devastating disease.

The Skin

Air bath therapy, one of the most potent exercises known, involves exposing our bodies to the omnipresent element of air. Since birth, we have been enveloped in this essential component of life, making it an integral part of our existence. Our skin, the body's largest organ, serves as a reflection of our innermost selves, representing our personality and psyche. It functions not only as a protective barrier but also as a vital organ in its own right, often referred to as the "second heart." This is due to its role in the immune system, endocrine system, and even its ability to mimic the functions of other organs, such as the kidney, lung, and digestive system.

The skin's significance becomes even more apparent in extreme situations, such as severe burns, where its condition can significantly impact a patient's prognosis. In cases of kidney failure, the skin plays a critical role in eliminating excess uric acid, a process that can be observed through the occurrence of uremic frost—a crystallized urea deposit found on the skin of those suffering from chronic kidney disease. This emphasizes the skin's role as a vital organ in maintaining homeostasis and overall health.

Furthermore, the skin is not merely a passive barrier; it actively interacts with its environment, responding to stimuli such as temperature changes and emotional experiences. Goosebumps, for instance, are a familiar reaction triggered by exposure to cold or emotional arousal, highlighting the skin's dynamic nature. Additionally, the skin acts as an immune organ, evidenced by the administration of vaccines through injection into the skin, underscoring its crucial role in protecting the body from pathogens.

Beyond its protective and regulatory functions, the skin also serves as a diagnostic tool, offering insights into an individual's health and well-being. In chronic degenerative diseases like cancer, the skin often exhibits a pale, anaemic appearance, reflecting the underlying disease process. Infectious diseases can also manifest in the skin, as seen in the case of stretch marks associated with certain conditions.

The skin's remarkable versatility is further demonstrated by its ability to absorb substances, allowing for the application of drugs and nutrients through patches and liposomes. This unique feature underscores the skin's multifaceted role as both a protective barrier and a conduit for therapeutic interventions.

Even though the skin is an important part of both health and sickness, there isn't a lot of information on how to keep it healthy. It's just as important for the skin to clean out the body as it is for the liver. We can improve liver health and general health as a whole by helping the skin detoxify. It was stressed by Dr. Max Gerson that the liver is an important part of the detoxification process and that cancer often starts after the liver stops working properly. A slow liver that can't get rid of toxins properly can cause dangerous substances to build up in the bloodstream, which is bad for cell health and body function as a whole.

This breakdown can make many organs not work right and weaken the immune system, making the body more likely to get illnesses from viruses, bacteria, and yeasts when they appear. When the redox potential of cells falls below what it should be, it can allow tumors and other dangerous growths to form. When this happens, the body becomes weak because its own abnormal cell growth goes against the natural order of life.

Carbon Monoxide

Carbon monoxide (CO) is a highly toxic gas that presents a significant danger to human well-being, frequently resulting in long-term diseases like cancer. Although it lacks visibility and scent, it can do severe harm to the body, especially when there is continuous exposure. The propensity of carbon monoxide (CO) to attach to hemoglobin is particularly worrisome, as it does so with a binding affinity that is 200 times stronger than that of oxygen. The reduced binding affinity of oxygen to cells hinders crucial cellular operations and may result in various health problems.

CO poisoning is particularly insidious since it can develop gradually, thereby impairing the body's natural functioning. Although rapid death can occur from acute exposure to high amounts of CO, chronic exposure to lower levels is as hazardous due to its potential to cause the development of cancer and other severe health disorders. The effect of carbon monoxide (CO) on the oxygenation of cells is extremely important. The body needs a considerably higher amount of oxygen to remove CO from hemoglobin, which worsens the problem even more.

Cancer is among the several outcomes of prolonged carbon monoxide exposure. The range of potential health concerns linked to carbon monoxide (CO) exposure is vast, encompassing chronic fatigue, memory impairments, work-related difficulties, sleep disturbances, dizziness, neurological diseases, paresthesia (abnormal sensations), recurring infections, gastrointestinal pain, and diarrhea. The wide array of symptoms emphasizes the extensive impact of carbon monoxide on the body's systems, emphasizing the immediate necessity to tackle this widespread health hazard.

Furthermore, aside from its immediate effects on well-being, carbon monoxide (CO) can also pose significant consequences for both the safety and efficiency of the workplace. Individuals who are exposed to elevated quantities of carbon monoxide (CO) may encounter a decline in cognitive abilities, diminished ability to make decisions, and a drop in overall performance. The implications of these effects can have significant impacts on both persons and organizations, underscoring the necessity of implementing steps to reduce exposure to carbon monoxide in professional environments.

Due to the severe health hazards linked to carbon monoxide (CO) exposure, it is imperative to adopt preventive measures to reduce the likelihood of poisoning. This entails guaranteeing enough airflow in enclosed areas, routinely inspecting and upkeeping gas devices, and incorporating carbon monoxide detectors in residential and occupational settings. By increasing public knowledge about the hazards of carbon monoxide and implementing suitable preventive measures, we may safeguard ourselves and those around us against this imperceptible threat.

The Airbath

The airbath is a tool and exercise that has multiple therapeutic benefits on the body, making it useful in the battle against cancer. A key factor in its effectiveness is its capacity to improve oxygenation. The significance of the airbath's influence is emphasized by the discoveries made by Otto Warburg about a century ago, which shown that tumors had a greater rate of glucose consumption in comparison to healthy tissues. Significantly, he observed that a substantial portion of the glucose eaten by tumors undergoes fermentation to produce lactate, rather than being oxidized by respiratory mechanisms. Furthermore, cancer is universally associated with cellular and tissue hypoxia, indicating that it is a state marked by a lack of oxygen.

The airbath's relevance rests in its capacity to mitigate these processes. The airbath provides the body with ample fresh air and oxygen, which can help counteract cellular hypoxia and potentially reverse the fermentation process. The presence of abundant oxygen in this environment produces an inhospitable setting for cancer cells, which flourish in sugar-fueled anaerobic conditions.

In addition, the airbath also enhances overall blood circulation. The airbath facilitates the circulation of sluggish venous blood from the skin back to the heart. Enhancing circulation in the skin, being one of the body's major organs, leads to enhanced circulation throughout the entire body. Improved blood flow aids in the elimination of toxins by promoting their expulsion through the skin. The airbath promotes cutaneous respiration and facilitates the elimination of toxins, hence reducing the workload on the liver and kidneys.

Another significant benefit of the airbath in the context of cancer therapy is its feasibility. It is universally accessible, irrespective of geographical location. The airbath can be conducted independently in one's own room, without requiring any support. The cost-effectiveness and simplicity of this option make it a practical choice for persons looking for complementary methods of treating cancer.

The airbath exercise is a powerful treatment for cancer because it increases oxygen levels, enhances blood flow, and aids in the removal of toxins. The ease of integration into one's daily routine, along with its cost-effectiveness, further amplifies its attractiveness as an adjunctive treatment for cancer.

Contrary to the simplistic approach of the airbath exercises proposed by Lehman and Lobrey, the Airbath method advocated by Nishi involves a more structured and systematic sequence of exercises. Lehman's method simply requires the patient to expose their naked body to fresh air for 15 to 20 minutes, while Lobrey's alternative involves covering and uncovering the body to stimulate venous return, which he refers to as "the second heart," aiding in general circulation. In contrast, Nishi's Airbath method incorporates a precise sequence of covering and exposing the body to fresh air, following a specific timing regimen facilitated by the use of a timer.

Nishi's Airbath is an alternating process that begins with covering the body and then exposing it to fresh air in a regulated manner. This sequence is crucial, as it helps optimize the benefits of the airbath. The use of a timer ensures that each phase of the airbath is carried out for the appropriate duration, maximizing its effectiveness.

The structured nature of Nishi's Airbath sets it apart from other methods, as it emphasizes the importance of following the timing and sequence in achieving optimal results. This approach reflects Nishi's holistic understanding of the body and its functions, highlighting the interconnectedness of various physiological processes.

Overall, Nishi's Airbath offers a comprehensive and methodical approach to harnessing the benefits of fresh air, highlighting the significance of proper timing and sequence in optimizing the therapeutic effects of the airbath.

The airbath of Nishi contains **11 cycles**. It is a sequence of being naked then clothed. The best way to do it is to wear a bathrobe so it is easier to take it to expose your body to fresh air.

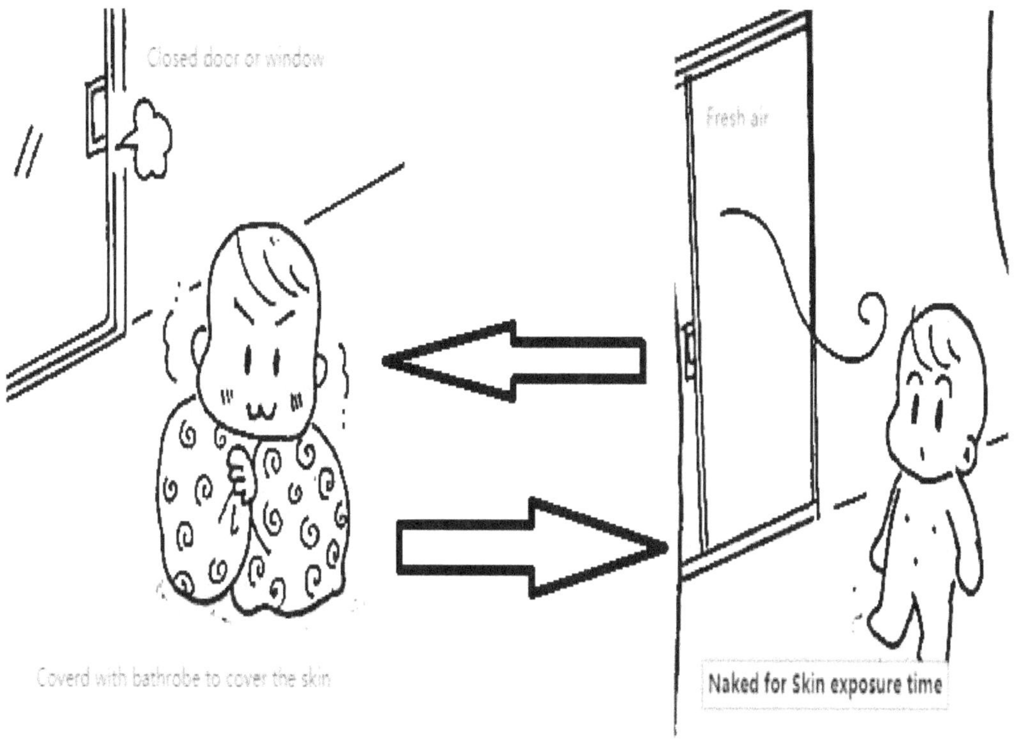
Closed door or window
Fresh air
Coverd with bathrobe to cover the skin
Naked for Skin exposure time

Cycles	Time being naked	Time being dressed
1	20 secs	1 minute
2	30	1 minute
3	40	1 minute
4	50	1 minute
5	60	1 minute and half
6	70	1 minute and half
7	80	1 minute and half
8	90	2 minutes
9	100	2 minutes
10	110	2 minutes
11	120	Rest on a hard floor dressed to stimulate the liver

Important note: The airbath needs to be done in a place exposed to

fresh air. You do not do it in a place with air pollution or around fumes.

The whole idea of the airbath is to expose the body to fresh air and burn carbon monoxide.

The airbath is free and can be used by anyone. For an invalid person, it can be done inside a room where the windows are wild open to allow fresh air to circulate.

For cancer prevention, performing the airbath exercise twice daily is sufficient. However, for individuals with chronic diseases like cancer, it is recommended to do the exercise at least 6 to 10 times a day. In more advanced cancer cases, increasing the frequency to 13 times a day may be beneficial. The exercise, though somewhat time-consuming, requires a minimum of 30 minutes to complete the entire sequence, but the health benefits make it worthwhile. For individuals with chronic carbon monoxide poisoning, the exercise should be done 4 to 6 times a day for at least 6 months, followed by twice daily as a preventive measure.

The airbath exercise is both refreshing and simple to perform. All that is needed is a bathrobe to cover oneself, which can be removed during the exposure to fresh air. It is essential to use common sense and perform the exercise in a clean area, avoiding industrial zones, places with air pollution, or environments with toxic gases. The primary purpose of the exercise is to utilize fresh air to cleanse both the sky and the body.

For those seeking a comprehensive approach to holistic cancer treatment, my book "The Four Elements of Nature Against Cancer" provides an in-depth protocol. This book offers detailed guidance on nutrition, supplements, and detoxification methods that can enhance treatment effectiveness.

Finally, the psyche of a cancer patient plays a crucial role in the healing process. Meditation can be incredibly beneficial in this regard, particularly during the healing journey and potential healing crises.

One simple yet effective method is to meditate for at least 40 minutes, sitting still and focusing solely on your breath with your eyes closed.

This practice can enhance the body's resilience and complement the benefits of the airbath exercise.

THE END